I0406790

Encyclopedia of Decoding DNA Sequence.

A Definitive Guide.

David Gomadza

First Global President of The World

www.twofuture.world

Encyclopedia of Decoding DNA Sequence. A Definitive Guide.

DEDICATION

A better future.

Table of Contents

Encyclopedia of Decoding DNA Sequence. A Definitive Guide.

ACKNOWLEDGMENTS

A Big Thanks to Tomorrow's World Order.

CHAPTER ONE

What is DNA?

DNA stands for Deoxyribonucleic acid.
DNA is a large molecule that carries genetic information, about the functioning, growth, and reproduction of all living organisms. It consists of a polynucleotide that bonds and binds together to form a double helix. DNA is essential for all living organisms.

The two DNA strands are known as polynucleotides as they are composed of simpler monomeric units called nucleotides. Each nucleotide is composed of one of four nitrogen-containing nucleobases (cytosine [C], guanine [G], adenine [A] or thymine [T]), a sugar called deoxyribose, and a phosphate group. The nucleotides are joined to one another in a chain by covalent bonds (known as the phosphodiester linkage) between the sugar of one nucleotide and the phosphate of the next, resulting in an alternating sugar-phosphate backbone. The nitrogenous bases of the two separate polynucleotide strands are bound together, according to base pairing rules (A with T and C with G), with hydrogen bonds to make double-stranded DNA. The complementary nitrogenous bases are divided into two groups, pyrimidines and purines. In DNA, the pyrimidines are thymine and cytosine; the purines are adenine and guanine.
Wikipedia

1

In short, DNA is a molecule that carries the genetic code of each person on earth, the code being unique to that person only.

20 Amino acids, their Number code, and their corresponding DNA codons

Amino Acid	Number Code	DNA codons
Isoleucine	12	ATT, ATC, ATA
Leucine	2	CTT, CTC, CTA, CTG, TTA, TTG
Valine	17	GTT, GTC, GTA, GTG
Phenylalanine	1	TTT, TTC
Methionine	13	ATG
Cysteine	6	TGT, TGC
Alanine	18	GCT, GCC, GCA, GCG
Glycine	21	GGT, GGC, GGA, GGG
Proline	8	CCT, CCC, CCA, CCG
Threonine	14	ACT, ACC, ACA, ACG
Serine	3	TCT, TCC, TCA, TCG, AGT, AGC
Tyrosine	4	TAT, TAC
Tryptophan	7	TGG
Glutamine	10	CAA, CAG
Asparagine	15	AAT, AAC
Histidine	9	CAT, CAC
Glutamic acid	20	GAA, GAG
Aspartic acid	19	GAT, GAC
Lysine	16	AAA, AAG
Arginine	11	CGT, CGC, CGA, CGG, AGA, AGG
Stop codons Stop	5	TAA, TAG, TGA
Pause		CCC

There are sixty-four possible 3-letter combinations of the DNA coding units Thymine T, Ardinine A, Cytosine C, and Guanine G.

I am going to use the bible to decode DNA sequences. I will use Ezekiel's vision.
Expanded in Chapter Five.

Ezekiel's Vision of God

1 Now it came to pass in the thirtieth year, in the fourth month, on the fifth day of the month, as I was among the captives by the River Chebar, that the heavens were opened and I saw visions[a] of God. 2 On the fifth day of the month, which was in the fifth year of King Jehoiachin's captivity, 3 the word of the LORD came expressly to Ezekiel the priest, the son of Buzi, in the land of the [b]Chaldeans by the River Chebar; and the hand of the LORD was upon him there.

*4 Then I looked, and behold, a whirlwind was coming out of the north, a great cloud with raging fire engulfing itself; and brightness was all around it and radiating out of its midst like the color of amber, out of the midst of the fire. 5 **Also from within it came the likeness of four living creatures.** And this was their appearance: they had the likeness of a man. 6 **Each one had four faces, and each one had four wings.** 7 Their [c]legs were straight, and the soles of their feet were like the soles of calves' feet. They sparkled like the color of burnished bronze. 8 The hands of a man were under their wings on their four sides; and each of the four had faces and wings. 9 Their wings touched one another. The creatures did not turn when they went, but each one went straight forward.*

*10 **As for the likeness of their faces, each had the face of a man; each of the four had the face of a lion on the right side, each of the four had the face of an ox on the left side, and each of the four had the face of an eagle.** 11 **Thus were their faces. Their wings stretched upward; two wings of each one touched one another, and two covered their bodies.** 12 And each one went straight forward; they went wherever the spirit wanted to go, and they did not turn when they went.*

13 As for the likeness of the living creatures, their appearance was like burning coals of fire, like the appearance of torches going back and forth among the living creatures. The fire was bright, and out of the fire went lightning. [14] *And the living creatures ran back and forth, in appearance like a flash of lightning.*

[15] ***Now as I looked at the living creatures, behold, a wheel was on the earth beside each living creature with its four faces.*** [16] *The appearance of the wheels and their workings was like the color of beryl, and all four had the same likeness.* ***The appearance of their workings was, as it were, a wheel in the middle of a wheel.*** [17] *When they moved, they went toward any one of four directions; they did not turn aside when they went.* [18] *As for their rims, they were so high they were impressive; and their rims were full of eyes, all around the four of them.* [19] ***When the living creatures went, the wheels went beside them; and when the living creatures were lifted from the earth, the wheels were lifted.*** [20] *Wherever the spirit wanted to go, they went, because there the spirit went; and the wheels were lifted together with them, for the spirit of the* [d]*living creatures was in the wheels.* [21] *When those went, these went; when those stood, these stood; and when those were lifted up from the earth, the wheels were lifted up together with them, for the spirit of the* [e]*living creatures was in the wheels.*

[22] ***The likeness of the*** [f]***firmament above the heads of the*** [g]***living creatures was like the color of an awesome crystal, stretched out over their heads.*** [23] *And under the firmament their wings spread out straight, one toward another. Each one had two which covered one side, and each one had two which covered the other side of the body.* [24] *When they went, I heard the noise of their wings, like the noise of many waters, like the voice of the Almighty, a tumult like the noise of an army; and when they stood still, they let down their wings.* [25] *A voice came from above the firmament that was over their heads; whenever they stood, they let down their wings.*

[26] *And above the firmament over their heads was the likeness of a throne, in appearance like a sapphire stone; on the likeness of the throne was a likeness with the appearance of a man high above it.* [27] *Also from the appearance of His waist and upward I*

saw, as it were, the color of amber with the appearance of fire all around within it; and from the appearance of His waist and downward I saw, as it were, the appearance of fire with brightness all around. [28] Like the appearance of a rainbow in a cloud on a rainy day, so was the appearance of the brightness all around it. This was the appearance of the likeness of the glory of the LORD.

New International Bible.

The DNA Sequence Rules.

A complete set of a function or trait must have 12 DNA sequence letters. Any three letters of any base can form a protein. The bases are Adenine A, Guanine G, Thymine T, and Cytosine C. A combination of any three of these can form a protein. To know which proteins, make up a trait or function of a body we must look at four connected occurrences at any time. The complete set of everything in nature has four ways. Just like the season they come in four different ways. The complete rotation of everything is depicted as a four-headed creature or being. As on earth as in heaven as in humans. Proteins are the building blocks of life. Even though you will have expected a 16 DNA sequence based on Ezekiel's vision, four creatures each with four heads. A protein can be identified and defined just by a combination of any three bases and not four bases. Therefore, any three combinations of either Adenine A, Cytosine C, Guanine G, and or Thymine T is enough to identify a protein.

We need four stages in total for each codon.

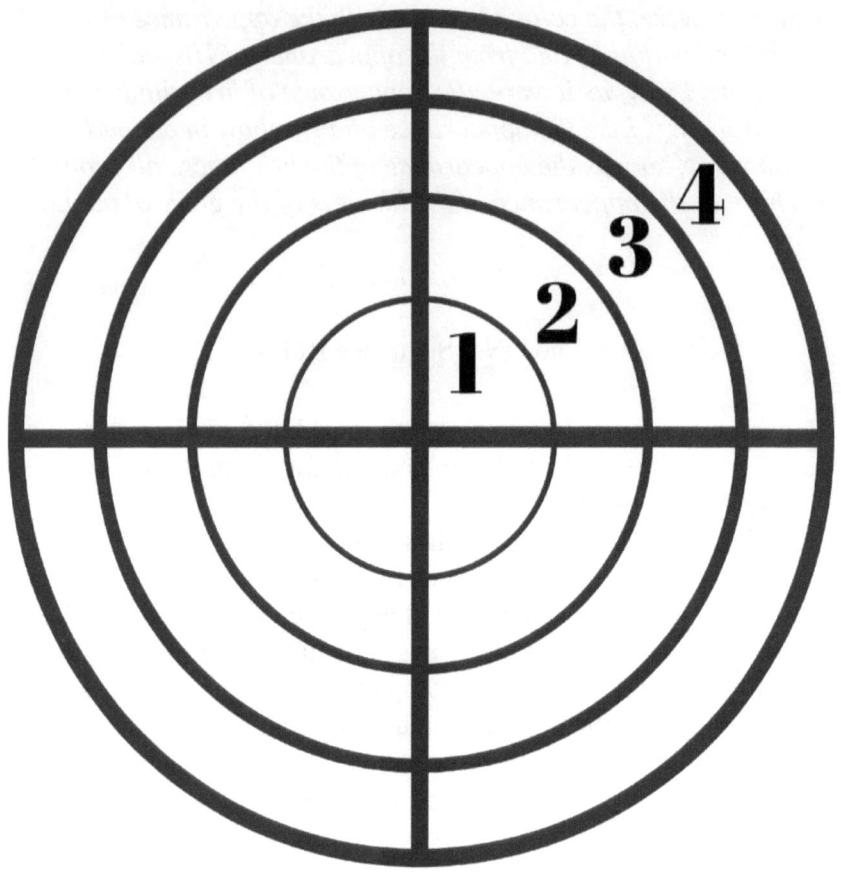

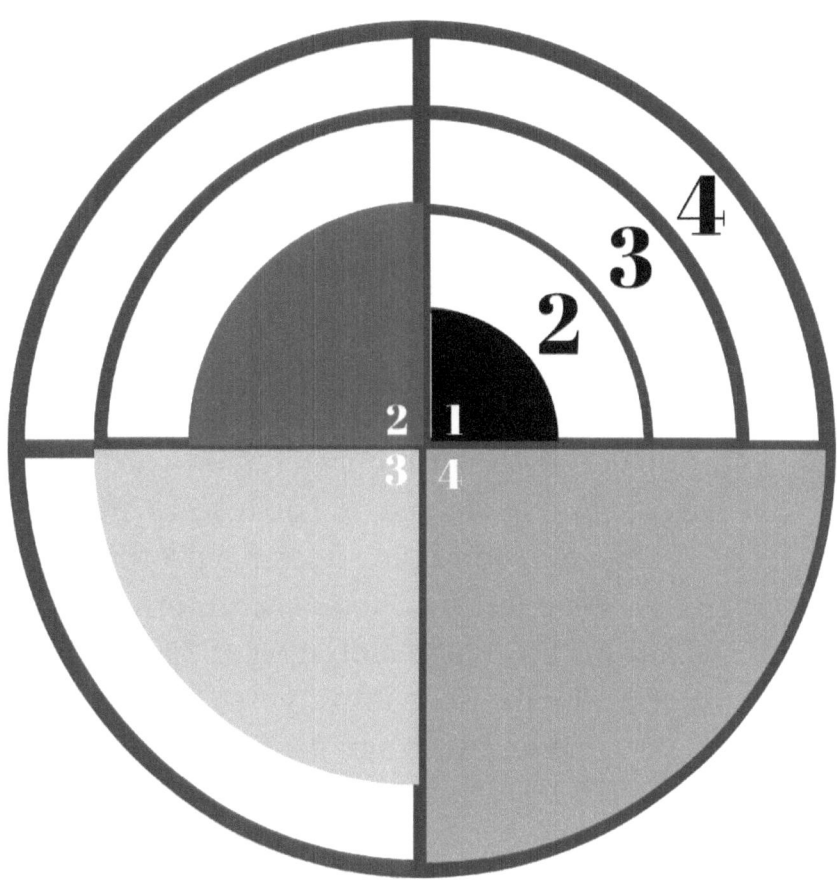

DNA Sequencing Patterns and Rules

The body arranges each function of the body or an attribute or trait or characteristic of a person as a 12-letter DNA sequence based on the four bases of DNA namely Adenine [A], Cytocine [C], Thymine [T] and Guanine [G].

It derives at the number 12 letter word DNA sequence based on the letters of DNA that can combine to form a protein that is three letters of bases can form a protein. The body then look at four cycles and join these four cycles to form a word for that trait.

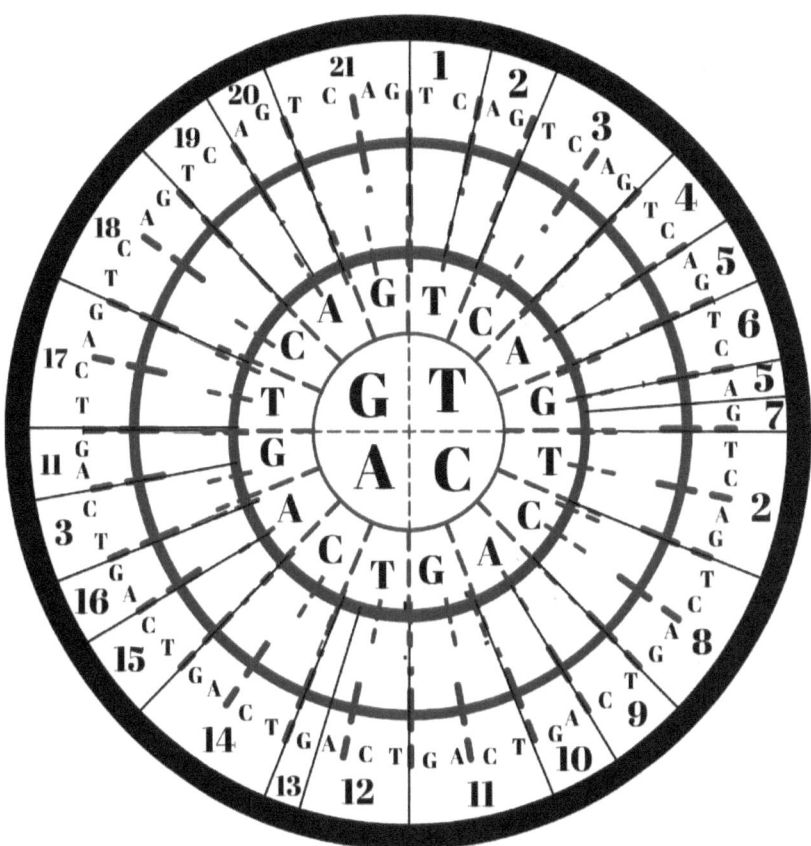

[16] *The appearance of the wheels and their workings was like the color of beryl, and all four had the same likeness.* **The appearance of their workings was, as it were, a wheel in the middle of a wheel.** [17] *When they moved, they went toward any one of four directions; they did not turn aside when they went.*

The man, lion, ox, and eagle are the base creature kingdoms each representing its kingdom namely; humans represented by the face of a man, wild animals represented by a lion, and domesticated animals represented by an ox while birds and flying creatures represented by the eagle. These correspond to the four bases in Adenine, Thymine, Cytosine and Guanine.

64 Possible Combinations.

There are sixty-four possible 3-letter combinations of the DNA coding units Thymine T, Ardinine A, Cytosine C and Guanine G.

Each creature had four heads and all four creatures had wings touching one another. The complete circle would mean four times four times four.

DNA Sequence Protein Combination Key

1	Phenylalanine
2	Leucine
3	Serine
4	Tyrosine
5	STOP
6	Cysteine
7	Tryptophan
8	Proline
9	Histidine
10	Glutamine
11	Arginine
12	Isoleucine
13	Methionine
14	Threonine
15	Asparagine
16	Lysine
17	Valine
18	Alanine
19	Aspartic Acid
20	Glutamic Acid
21	Glycine

DNA as a language or like a language.

Like I said at the beginning, DNA is like a manual for instructions to make proteins. Any written instructions are through a language that has rules for encoding that language so that it is understood.

That means DNA has a Start, a Pause, and a Stop.

Start of a DNA Sequence.

A start is the beginning of a DNA sequence.
Usually starts with an A [Adenine] and ends with a T [Thymine].
It does not matter what it is between.
Start can be as simple as A_T
It is true also that the start can be any of the following.
ACT for a male or ACC for a female.
AAT for a male and AAC for a female DNA. AGT for a male
DNA and AAC for a female DNA.

Pause of a DNA Sequence.

Just like a language, the DNA sequence has a pause as a brief stop.
This is represented by three Cytosines. Therefore, a Pause is CCC.

Stop of a DNA sequence.

Just like a language. A stop depicts when to stop in the sequence to
start something new. A stop can be at any stage in the sequence but
after Tyrosine or Cysteine.
A stop sequence can be any of the following.
AAA
ATG
GTA.

The left-hand thumb finger is the starting point.

When the body starts compiling a body's DNA it always starts
from the left hand's thumb finger. This is the starting point.

End of a DNA sequence.

The body will end the DNA sequence with a CCC first. You know from above that this is a pause.

Then followed by a Start.
You also know that a Start can be any of these.
AAT for a male and AAC for a female.
GTG is a start for DNA sequence that involves all animals and is
never used as a start for human DNA.
ATT is used for starting DNA for flying birds and not for humans.
TAT for a male or TAC for a female.
ACT for a male or ACC for a female.

Then followed by a STOP but only this stop is used at the end of
any DNA sequence as this means the real end.
GTA.

The body compiles and updates a person's DNA several times
throughout life.
First DNA at birth.
The body compiles the person's DNA at birth.
CTCTCTCTCTCT
This DNA sequence is also referred to as God or sometimes life.

DNA is compiled every year, also on birthdays.

This DNA sequence CTCTCTCTCTCT divided by a person's age
gives an aggregate life DNA index that can be used to determine
the well-being of a person. It can also be used to calculate a
person's lifespan guide, etc.

The body calculates, compiles, and updates a person's DNA every
4 years.

Last day of compiling DNA.

The last body activity just before death is the calculation and
compilation of DNA.
The last DNA entry before air exits the body is a
GTAGTAGTAGTA

Therefore, GTAGTAGTAGTA is DEATH.

CHAPTER TWO

How does the body compile a person's DNA and how does it do it?

A body can easily produce a long chain of DNA sequences consisting of fifty-two billion two hundred elements of the four bases namely Adenine A, Cytosine C, Guanine G, and or Thymine T for a normal person. This can be a long chain, but the body can tell any part within the chain. This is because the body has an order of creating this DNA sequence. So, it will simply calculate position even though this might not be specific for every person.

It is interesting to note that the human DNA sequence of a normal person consists of more than 52 billion combinations in total. God's DNA has 53 billion and 600 combinations. Somehow when I time-travelled back to the past my DNA has become 53 billion 600 as well. I wore God's stencil, just not sure if this is temporary or not. Out of this world experience. See last chapter for further reading references.

The body follows a specific pattern and rules to compile a human DNA sequence.

The body follows its rules to produce an individual's DNA sequence.

Recap of some of the rules I mentioned above.
1. The opening DNA sequence at birth is CTCTCTCTCTCT.
This is the same DNA sequence for GOD or Yahweh in Hebrew.
The start of life and everything.
Changing the last two letters with CC for a woman and with GA for a man gives the DNA sequence of people just birth.
Notice that since humans are created in God's image they must match.
Therefore, at birth, everyone is as good as God as they are God's image.
GOD or Yahweh's DNA sequence is CTCTCTCTCTCT.
For a woman at birth, it is CTCTCTCTCTCC.
For a man at birth, it is CTCTCTCTCTGA.
This is the starting point of a person's DNA at birth.

Proof of God in DNA
GOD or Yahweh's DNA sequence is
CTCTCTCTCTCT=2+3+2+3= leucine + serine + leucine + serine

Do you know that a human being has twenty-three chromosomes out of forty-six?

2. Four possible START of a DNA sequence are:
a] AAT for a male or AAC for a female.
b] CAT for a male or CAA for a female.
c] ACT for a male or ACC for a female.
d] TAT for a male or TAC for a female.
3. Female DNA sequence will always start with a CCT
4. Male DNA sequences will always start with a GTT.
5. The DNA sequence of a function or trait will always have twelve letters of the bases namely Adenine A, Cytosine C, Guanine G, and Thymine T.
6. The DNA sequence will always have a START, a PAUSE, and an end that is a STOP. Whereas CCC is a pause. A stop sequence can be any of the following: AAA, ATG, or a GTA.

7. The body will always read and compile DNA sequences from the left side of the body, specifically from the left thumb.

8. The body distinguishes between sexes and where body parts are governed by a person's sex the body asks itself the sex of the individual concerned. A perfect example is when it reaches the nipples. These are both on males' and females' bodies. So, it must add another entry to the DNA about the sex of the individual.

9. The body distinguishes between the inside and outside of the body. Some parts and at some stage during compilation it look at inside parts for example at the inside spine, stomach, throat, head, etc. as distinguished from outside of the body.

10. The body looks at full body features and categorizes these. It looks at all organs and categories these. It then looks at specific points on the body although not in the order I am mentioning them here. Then it looks at compiling a toe-to-head DNA sequence. Then look at specific head parts, the nose, eyes, lips, teeth, hair, etc.

At some points, the body then looks at all orifices on the body namely, anus, mouth, nostrils, ears, eyes, penis, and vagina.

11. The body looks at defective orifices. Extra orifices induced by body defects like a second opening somewhere it should not be.

12. The body will look also at the inside. The factors that determine things like height, lifespan, age-related deaths, family tree, etc. The body will calculate the aggregate life index where it takes DNA sequence at birth CTCTCTCTCTCT and divide this by the age of a person.

Above 0 means great. The body also looks at other function parameters like breathing.

The body will calculate an overall score.

After all this, the body completes and ends the DNA sequence first with a pause which is a CCC. Then with a START which can either be AAT for a male or AAC for a female, ATT is used to denote the start of DNA for flying birds and is never used as a start for human DNA. Or ACT for a male or an ACC for a female. Then the end of the DNA sequence is shown by a GTA only which is a STOP specific for ending the DNA sequence.

13. Therefore when a person dies the last DNA sequence entry will be GTAGTAGTAGTA.

CHAPTER THREE

The Actual Process the Body Uses to Compile a Person's DNA.
A Step-by-Step Definitive Guide.
Initial starting point.
Left-hand thumb finger.

But I explained in the previous chapter that the body when
compiling DNA distinguishes between males and females.
Also, recall that I said the initial entry at birth of any person is the
LIFE DNA sequence which is CTCTCTCTCTCT.

Starting DNA for females is the following.
We remove the last two parts of the sequence of God and add CC
at the end of the God. This shows that this DNA is female that is
for a female.
Therefore, CC denotes women.

Therefore, the START DNA sequence for a female will be.
CTCTCTCTCTCC

Starting DNA for males is the following.

We remove the last two parts of the sequence of LIFE and add a
GA at the end of this LIFE sequence. This shows that this DNA is

for a male. Therefore, GA denotes a male.
Therefore, the START of a DNA sequence is CTCTCTCTCTGA.

Starting point of any DNA Sequence.

1. The left-hand thumbs.

Females is CTCTCTCTCTCC
Males is CTCTCTCTCTGA

2. The left-hand Index finger is the second place DNA is compiled for.
The Female left hand index finger is GTAGTCGCCTCC.
Male left hand index finger is CTCTGGCTCCGA.

3. The left-hand Middle finger is the third point where DNA is compiled for.
Female left hand middle finger DNA sequence is.
GTACCTATATCC.
Male left hand middle finger DNA sequence is.
CTCTCCGTAGGA

4. The left-hand ring finger is the fourth place DNA sequence is compiled for.
Female left hand ring finger DNA sequence is.
GTGTCCTAGACC
The male's left hand ring finger DNA sequence is.
CTCTCCGATCGA

5. The left-hand little finger is the fifth place DNA is compiled for.
Female left hand little finger is.
GTGTCTATGTCC
Male left hand little finger is.
CTCCGAGATCGA

Therefore, I can say that the female DNA sequence will start as follows.

Female left-hand thumb + Female left-hand index finger + Female left-hand middle finger + Female left-hand ring finger + Female left-hand little finger.

CTCTCTCTCTCC + GTAGTCGCCTCC + GTACCTATATCC + GTGTCCTAGACC + GTGTCTATGTCC

= female left-hand fingers DNA sequence

This is equal to:
CTCTCTCTCTCCGTAGTCGCCTCCGTACCTATATCC GTGTCCTAGACCGTGTCTATGTCC.

A male's starting DNA sequence is the starting DNA sequence from his left-hand thumb to the left-hand little finger. I explained above that all male DNA sequences for every part end with GA. Therefore, let us compile this DNA from the above information.

Male's starting DNA sequence.

Male left hand thumb + Male left hand index finger + Male left hand middle finger + Male left hand ring finger + Male left hand little finger
= CTCTCTCTCTGA + CTCTGGCTCCGA + CTCTCCGTAGGA + CTCTCCGATCGA + CTCCGAGATCGA
= Male's left hand fingers DNA sequence

This is equal to.
CTCTCTCTCTGACTCTGGCTCCGACTCTCCGTAGG ACTCTCCGATCGACTCCGAGATCGA.

Start of a DNA sequence.

In the first chapter, I mentioned that there are four possible starts to a DNA sequence.
2. Four possible START of a DNA sequence are:
a] AAT for male or AAC for female.

b] CAT for male or CAA for female.
c] ACT for male or ACC for female.
d] TAT for a male and TAC for a female.

Therefore, depending on other factors, I will explain in later chapters. The possible start for a female DNA sequence might include.

AAC +
CTCTCTCTCTCCGTAGTCGCCTCCGTACCTATATCC
GTGTCCTAGACCGTGTCTATGTCC.

This can be.
AACCTCTCTCTCTCCGTAGTCGCCTCCGTACCTATA
TCCGTGTCCTAGACCGTGTCTATGTCC.

As such a male DNA sequence can be
AAT +
CTCTCTCTCTGACTCTGGCTCCGACTCTCCGTAGG
ACTCTCCGATCGACTCCGAGATCGA.

This can be.
AATCTCTCTCTCTGACTCTGGCTCCGACTCTCCGTA
GGACTCTCCGATCGACTCCGAGATCGA

DNA sequence for a female can start with an ACC making the start of female DNA sequence be.

ACCCTCTCTCTCTCCGTAGTCGCCTCCGTACCTATA
TCCGTGTCCTAGACCGTGTCTATGTCC.

Likewise, a male DNA sequence can start with ACT. That makes the DNA sequence be.
ACTCTCTCTCTCTGACTCTGGCTCCGACTCTCCGTA
GGACTCTCCGATCGACTCCGAGATCGA

Recap the chapter.

The body compiles DNA sequences starting from the left hand of a person, namely from the left-hand thumb finger.
Since the start is the same as God CTCTCTCTCTCT this is usually the first entry differentiated by sex.

Therefore, the beginning is.
CTCTCTCTCTCT
Which is the same as God or Yahweh.

Then the body asks for the sex [whether male or female.]
If male remove the last two letters and replace them with a GA.

If female, then remove the last two letters and replace them with a CC.

But just like any written language, there are rules for writing the language. There are several starts.
Therefore, before even the life stage CTCTCTCTCTCT, there are opening letters that must be introduced at the beginning.

DNA sequence construction rules.

The possible STARTs of any DNA.
Sex? [Male or female]

Possible START if male.

1. AAT
2. TAT
3. ACT
4. CAT

Possible START if female.

1. AAC
2. TAC
3. ACC
4. CAA

There are other possible STARTs to a DNA and these involve animals and flying birds.

1. GTG is a start for DNA sequence that involves all animals and never used as a start for human DNA.
2. ATT is used for starting DNA for flying birds and not for humans.

The body compiles DNA sequences following a particular order.

These are the first steps. Step by step.

1. Opening START
2. +
3. Left hand thumb hand. This is the same as the DNA of life CTCTCTCTCTCT.
4. If a female add a CC at the end after removing the last two letters. If male remove the last two letters and add GA.
5. +
6. Left hand Index finger.
7. +
8. Left hand Middle finger.
9. +
10. Left hand Ring finger.
11. +
12. Left hand little finger.

Brace up and buckle up because we are now going deeper. Way too deep with this DNA. I will now give you the step-by-step sequence the body uses to compile the DNA and its length. I will then look at the examples. To go about this as we did above where I calculate the actual DNA of every part of the body, the function or traits is way too complicated and might require a book of its own. Therefore, I will list the DNA sequence without the actual values first. Then calculate the values as we go. But I think it is interesting to find out how the body compiles this DNA sequence.

At first, it seemed like rocket science. But just remember it is just like the language we speak. It is based on rules. Master the rules then you will be able to calculate the needed values easily.
Anything without knowing its construction rules, etc. is cumbersome. But know the rules and it becomes information at your fingertips.
Are you ready?
Let us go. I will show you everything about DNA sequencing.

CHAPTER FOUR

DNA Sequencing. Exactly how the body does it. A step-by-step guide.
I will list all stages in order just as words without any arrows, etc.
Any word below the one above means this is the next stage after the above word. Unless they are explanations. Or sometimes the body has more information whether it is a female or male. Or whether it is inside of the body or outside etc.

HOW THE BODY COMPILES THE DNA SEQUENCE.

DNA Sequence START
Sex? Male or Female.
Possible START if male.

AAT
TAT
ACT
CAT

Possible START if female.

AAC
TAC
ACC
CAA

+

Left hand Thumb [LIFE=CTCTCTCTCTCT]

Sex [Male or Female]

If Male=CTCTCTCTCTGA

If Female =CTCTCTCTCTCC

+

Left hand Index finger.

+

Left hand Middle finger.

+

Left hand Ring finger.

+

Left hand little finger.

+

Left hand Elbow.

+

Left hand shoulder.

+

Left side armpit.

+

Left side hip bone.

+

Left side knee.

+

Left side calf.

+

Left side ankle.

+

Left side small toe.

+

Left side second toe.

+

Left side third toe.

+

Left side fourth toe.

+

Left side big toe.

+

Middle of left leg between heel and big toe.

+

Left side heel.

+

Left side calf.

+

Left side leg joint.

+

Lower buttocks.

+

Left buttock.

+

Anus

+

Scrotum

+

Left testicle.

+

Right testicle

+

Penis

+

Pubic region.

+

Naval

+

Center chest.

+

Left nipple.

+

Heart.

+

Right lung

+

Right nipple

+

Right armpit

+

Right elbow

+

Wrist joint

+

Little finger

+

Ring finger

+

Middle finger

+

Index finger

+

Thumb finger

+

Right Wrist

+

Right elbow

+

Right shoulder top

+

Right neck

+

Back center back

+

Back spine

+

Lumbar bone spine

+

Anus

+

Inside now through the anus

+

Inner back spine.

+

Inner top spine

+

Inner top neck

+

The Inner back head limbic system

+

Back head inside

+

Inside top head

+

Inside forehead

+

Middle of eyes groove

+

Nose bridge

+

Nose tip

+

Nose separator that separates nostrils.

+

Middle top lip.

+

Middle of closed lip

+

Lower lip bottom.

+

Middle chin

+

Middle throat.

+

Then all body parts.
Which includes the following.
Heart

+

Liver

+

Spleen

+

Diaphragm

+

Lung

+

Brain

+

Typhoid Gland

+

Heart

+

Blood

+

Skin

+

Hair

+

Nose

+

Eyes

+

Fingers

+

Toes

+

Nails

+

Lips

+

Eyebrows

+

Lip bottom

+

Lip top

+

Chin

+

Left eye.

+

Right eye

+

Neck

+

Outside of Thyroid gland
+
Sex? Female or Male
+
Middle center chest
+
Sex? Female or male
+
Nipples
+
Sex? Male or Female
+
Ovaries
Sex? Male=testicles female=ovaries
Fallopian tubes
Sex? Male =testicle tubes or for female fallopian tubes
Anus
Sex? Female = sex organs male= excretion.
+
Genitals.
Sex? Female or mal
+
Legs
Sex? Male or female
+
Calves
Sex? Female or male
+
Ankles
+
Heel
+
Bottom of foot
+
Nails
Sex? Female or male
+
Toes
+

Full body DNA sequence

+

Toes to head

+

Front to back.

+

Sex? Female or male

+

Hair
Sex? Male or female

+

Smile

+

Nose

+

Eyes; -
color
Widening
Sleepy
Drowsiness
Blindness
Water content
Crying
Laughing
Sneezing
What happens to your eyes when breathing?
Roundness
Sharp
Blinking
Sleeping
Mother
Father
Child
All children.

+

Forehead; -
Wrinkle pattern
Tightness
When thinking

When eyes open
Hairline
Roundness
+

Ears; -
Shape
Sliding with the head
Roundness
Grooves
Hearing
Surrounding effects.
+

Mouth; -
Wideness
Lip size
Plumpness
Wide shape?
Soft shape
+

Teeth: -
Whiteness
Spacing
Shape when breathing hard.
Rough
Fragility
+

Nose shape; -
Shape
Pointiness
Opening when breathing
Sensitivity to air. Smell and touch
Fragility
+

Forehead
+

Back head
+

Neck back
+

Chest front

+

Back spine

+

Naval abdomen

+

Back lumbar bone

+

Groin front

+

Anus back

+

Inside Spine

+

Inside Abdomen

+

Inside back spine

+

Inside the middle of the chest

+

Inside top back

+

Inside voice box

+

Sex? Male or female

+

Back neck back

+

Inside chin

+

Inside lip bottom

+

Inside back head hairline

+

Inside nose tip

+

Inside back head

+

Inside middle of the eyes

+

Inside back top head

+

Inside forehead

+

Inside the top of the head.

+

Middle of the throat as viewed from the top.

+

Arms

+

Sex? Female or male

+

Left arm.

+

Right arm

+

Sex organs hair
Sex? Male or female

+

Orifices

+

Anus
Sex? Female or male. Female sex organs.

+

Mouth

+

Nostrils
Position? Left or right.

+

Ears
Position? Left or right.

+

Eyes
Position? Left or right; -
Blinking
Watery
Sharpness

+

Penis

+

Vagina

+

Orifices due to defects if any?
Extra organs orifices?
Sex? Male or Female.

+

Insides

+

Height

+

Lifespan

+

Age-related deaths

+

Family tree.

+

Lifestyle

+

Blank if below 18 years.
Above 18 years use if the aggregate initial DNA
CTCTCTCTCTCT in relation to the age of the person.
Every year on birth body checks and updates DNA
Every four years the body updates DNA as well.

+

Organs
The body checks organ function in relation to age, etc.

+

Breathing.
The body checks overall breathing in relation to age. Looking at breathing as a function and all related factors.

+

The body now gives a score of health and function status of the body just before closing the DNA sequence.

+

Ends the DNA sequence first by putting a PAUSE which is a CCC.

+

This is followed by either a START which can be either an AAT, or an ACT for males, or their counterparts for females meaning an AAC or ACC.

+

Followed by a STOP that denotes the end of the DNA sequence which is a GTA.

The end of a full DNA sequence is sex sensitive as well.

GTA is the only definitive end to a DNA sequence but in this case the body would still ask for the sex.
So, this will be like the following.

End of DNA sequence.
GTA
Sex? Males add GA at the end. Females add a CC.
This will be like.
End of female DNA sequence=
GTACC

The end of a DNA sequence of a male would be like this.
GTAGA

CHAPTER FIVE

Now let us look at the possible protein combinations that are depicted from the twelve-letter DNA sequence the body uses and categorizes all activities, functions, traits, inside, organs, etc. The body names every function of a body as a twelve letter DNA sequence based on all four bases namely, Cytosine C, Guanine G, Adenine A, and Thymine T. The body names and places the twelve letter DNA sequences in the body for easy access.

Function or intended result and the twelve letter DNA sequence.

Blue eyes   in females = CTATGTCCGACC

                       In males =   CTATCATCGAGA

                       In animals = CTATACGTAGTA

Height   CTCCCGATCCCG

Weight   CCCTGAGGTTAT

Hair   CCATGCATGACT

Female breast growth   CTATCAGTTATA

Encyclopedia of Decoding DNA Sequence. A Definitive Guide.

Penis		CTTAGATACTTA
Penis growth in puberty		GGGTGATATTG
Penis growth in adults		GGGTGATACGT
Normal human growth		CTGTATAGTATG
Female breast growth during puberty		CTATTGATCTGA
Rejuvenating		CTATAGGATGTA
Aging		CCCTATACCGTA
Death		CCCTTTAAAGGG
Life		CTCTAAACCGTA
Eyes	female	CTCTGGATGACC
	Male	GTGTCCATCAGA
Blue eyes	female	CTGAGTGACTCC
	Male	CTGAGACGGA
Heart	Male	GTCCTAGACCGA
	Female	CTCCTAGGCCCC
Blood		GATCTCCTCTCT
Lungs	Female	GAGATCGAGGCC
	Male	CCGATCCCGAGA
Hair	Female	CCTCGAGTCCCC
	Male	GAGATCCTGGGA
Longevity		CTCTGACTCTCT

Encyclopedia of Decoding DNA Sequence. A Definitive Guide.

Life at birth	CTCTCTCTCTCT
God	CTCTCTCTCTCT

Left hand elbow	Female CTCTGACCTCCC
	Male GACTCTGATCGA

Left hand shoulder	Female GATCTCCCGACC
	Male CCTCCCCATCGA

Left side armpit	Female GATATCGGGACC
	Male CCTAGCGGTAGA

Left side hipbone	Female GATACCGACCCC
	Male GATATAGACCGA

Left knee	Female GATCGACCTCCC
	Male CCTAGGTACCGA

Left calf	Female GATCCCCGACC
	Male CTCTGACCGAGA

Left ankle	Female GATATACCGGCC
	Male CCTAGGCCTAGA

Left little toe	Female GGGAGCGCCCC
	Male GACCCCTAGAGA

Left leg second toe	Female GGGCTATTCCCC
	Male GGTATCTCCCGA

| Left leg third toe | Female CCCGTACCGTCC |

	Male GGGACGCCGAGA
Left leg fourth toe	Female CGGAGAGGTCCC
	Male GAGGTCTCGAGA
Left leg big toe	Female GAGAGATCTCCC
	Male CCCTGAGGGCGA
Anus	Male GGGCTCCATAGA

Anus for females is under sex organs. To confirm later how the body deals with this in DNA sequencing.

Recap.

The body names every function of the body, organs, etc. using a twelve letter DNA sequence name using the four base code letters namely Adenine A, Cytosine C, Guanine G, and Thymine T.

The body differentiates between sexes using CC for female and GA for males.

Therefore, in most cases, any sequence that ends in CC refers to women or something associated with women. GA is everything associated with males.

Now we want to convert this twelve letter DNA sequence name to its protein equivalent. This is because this code is an instruction manual given to make proteins. So, let us find out what proteins each name represents and try to find proof in the real world.

The underlying belief here is that every organ or function, or trait is influenced, or was made by a combination of these proteins. If we know what proteins were used to make these attributes in the first place, then replacing these proteins will strengthen that attribute or function as a repair function to restore that attribute or function.

This is what I call opening the blueprint of life.

What is the left and right of the north?

When one faces the rising sun, the back faces the west, the left hand represents the northern side, and the right hand represents the southern side.

Ezekiel's Vision of God.

[4] Then I looked, and behold, **a whirlwind was coming out of the north**, a great cloud with raging fire engulfing itself; and brightness *was* all around it and radiating out of its midst like the color of amber, out of the midst of the fire. [5] **Also from within it** *came* **the likeness of four living creatures.** And this *was* their appearance: they had the likeness of a man. [6] **Each one had four faces, and each one had four wings.** [7] Their [c]legs *were* straight, and the soles of their feet *were* like the soles of calves' feet. They sparkled like the color of burnished bronze. [8] The hands of a man *were* under their wings on their four sides; and each of the four had faces and wings. [9] Their wings touched one another. *The creatures* did not turn when they went, but each one went straight forward.

[15] Now as I looked at the living creatures, behold, a wheel *was* on the earth beside each living creature with its four faces. **[16]** The appearance of the wheels and their workings *was* like the color of beryl, and all four had the same likeness. **The appearance of their workings *was,* as it were, a wheel in the middle of a wheel.**

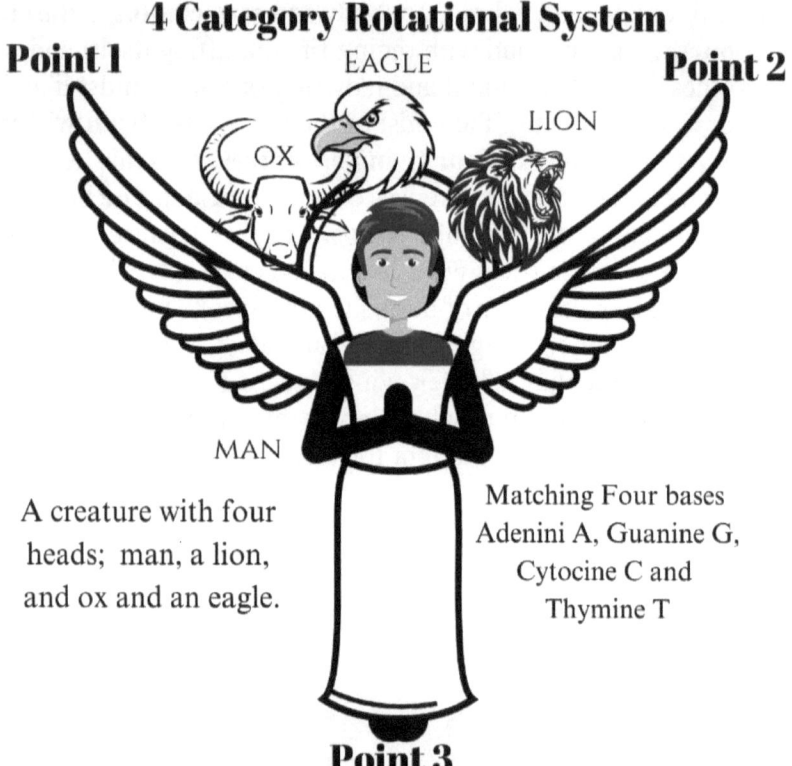

4 Category Rotational System

Point 1

EAGLE

Point 2

OX

LION

MAN

A creature with four heads; man, a lion, and ox and an eagle.

Matching Four bases Adenini A, Guanine G, Cytocine C and Thymine T

Point 3

3 Point System within a 4 rotation pattern

4 Category Rotational System

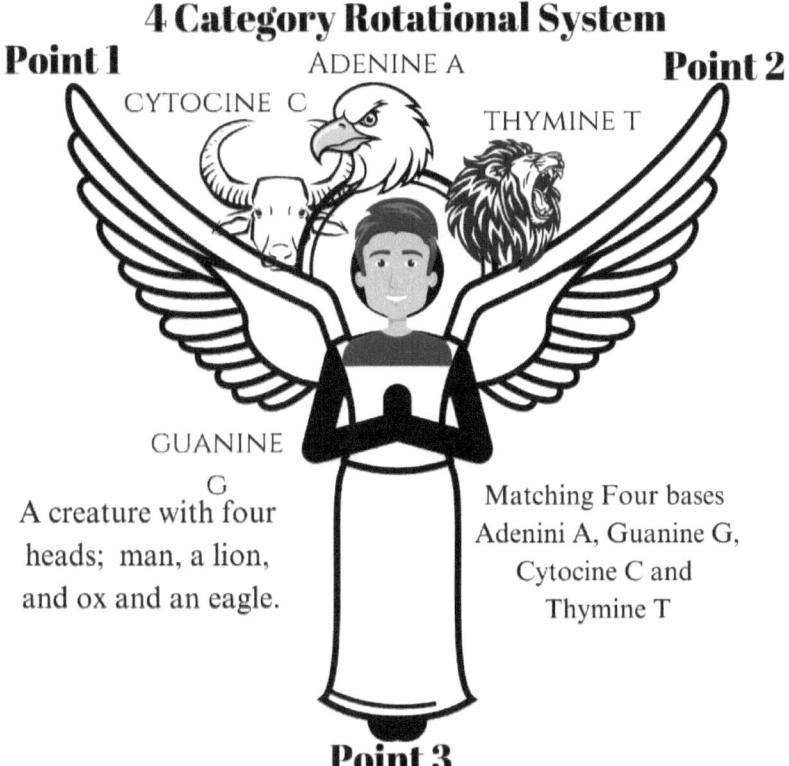

Point 1

ADENINE A

CYTOCINE C

THYMINE T

Point 2

GUANINE

G

A creature with four heads; man, a lion, and ox and an eagle.

Matching Four bases Adenini A, Guanine G, Cytocine C and Thymine T

Point 3

3 Point System within a 4 rotation pattern

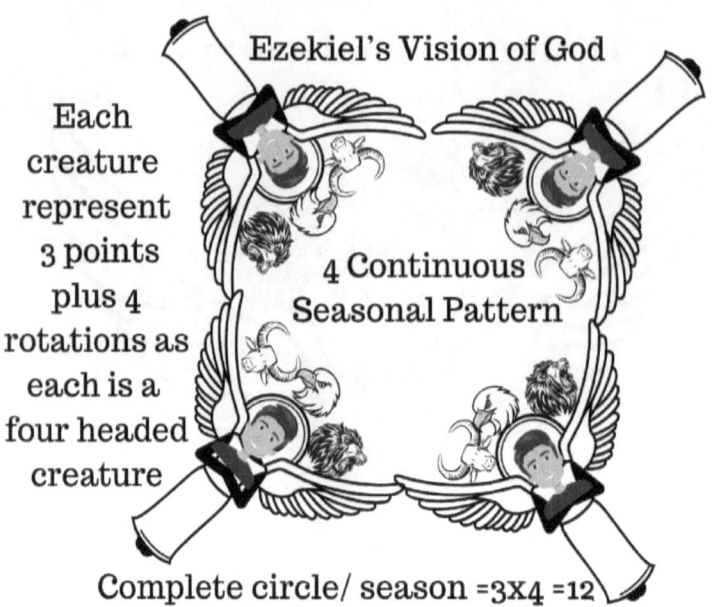

Ezekiel's Vision of God

Each creature represent 3 points plus 4 rotations as each is a four headed creature

4 Continuous Seasonal Pattern

Complete circle/ season =3x4 =12

5 Also from within it came the likeness of four living creatures. And this was their appearance: they had the likeness of a man. 6 Each one had four faces, and each one had four wings. 7 **Their [c]legs were straight, and the soles of their feet were like the soles of calves' feet**. They sparkled like the color of burnished bronze. 8 The hands of a man were under their wings on their four sides; and each of the four had faces and wings. **9 Their wings touched one another. The creatures did not turn when they went, but each one went straight forward.**

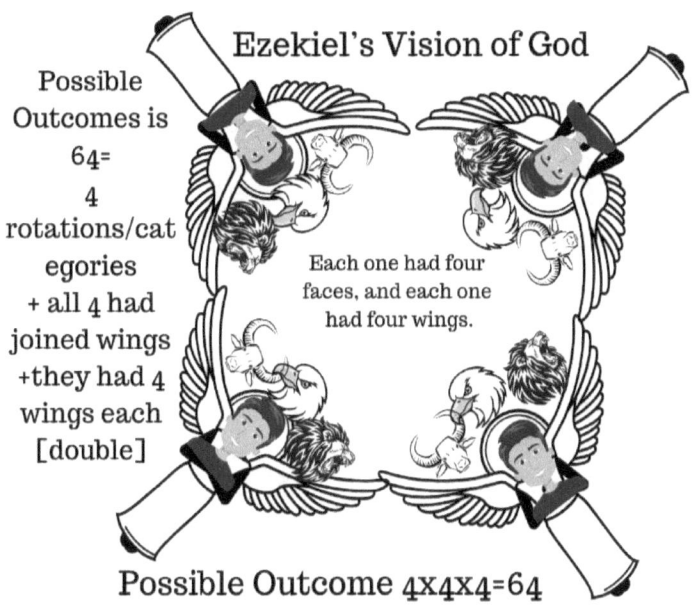

Ezekiel's Vision of God

Possible Outcomes is 64=
4 rotations/categories
+ all 4 had joined wings
+they had 4 wings each
[double]

Each one had four faces, and each one had four wings.

Possible Outcome 4x4x4=64

6 Each one had four faces, and each one had four wings...

9 Their wings touched one another. [They had 4 wings each meaning they can touch each other]

The creatures did not turn when they went, but each one went straight forward.

Ezekiel's Vision of God

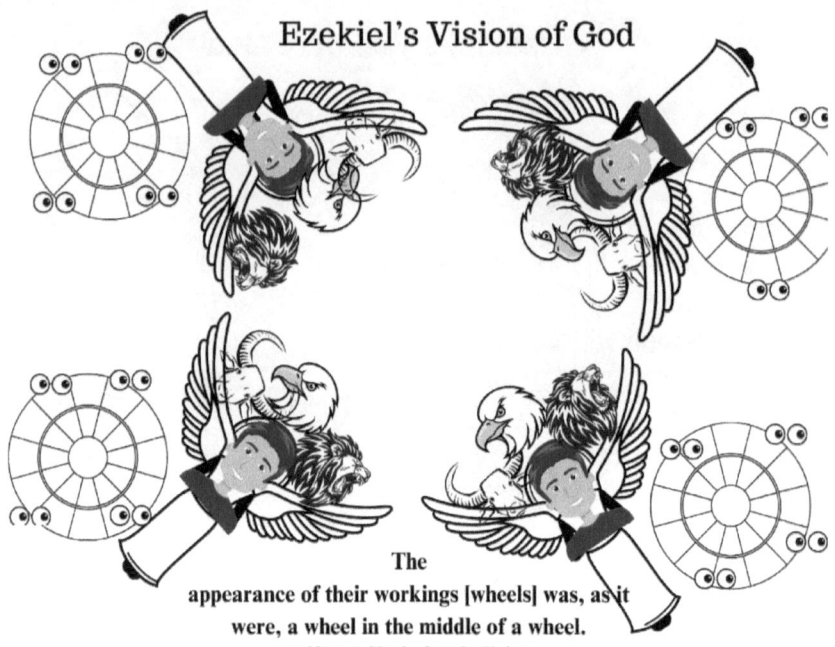

The appearance of their workings [wheels] was, as it were, a wheel in the middle of a wheel.

15 Now as I looked at the living creatures, behold, a wheel was on the earth beside each living creature with its four faces. 16 The appearance of the wheels and their workings was like the color of beryl, and all four had the same likeness. The appearance of their workings was, as it were, a wheel in the middle of a wheel.

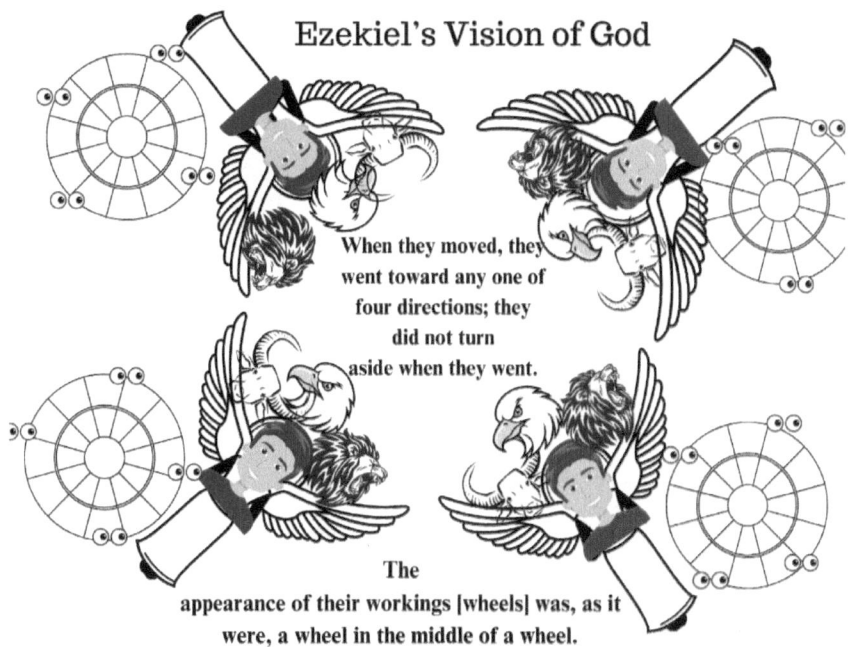

Ezekiel's Vision of God

When they moved, they went toward any one of four directions; they did not turn aside when they went.

The appearance of their workings [wheels] was, as it were, a wheel in the middle of a wheel.

As for their rims, they were so high they were awesome; and their rims were full of eyes, all around the four of them.

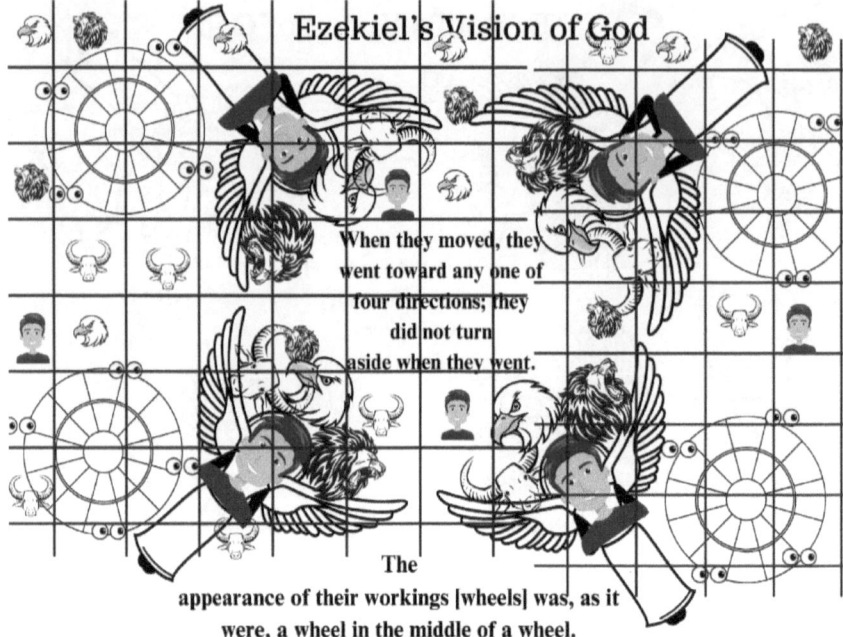

Ezekiel's Vision of God

When they moved, they went toward any one of four directions; they did not turn aside when they went.

The appearance of their workings [wheels] was, as it were, a wheel in the middle of a wheel.

The likeness of the [f]firmament above the heads of the [g]living creatures was like the color of an awesome crystal, stretched out over their heads.

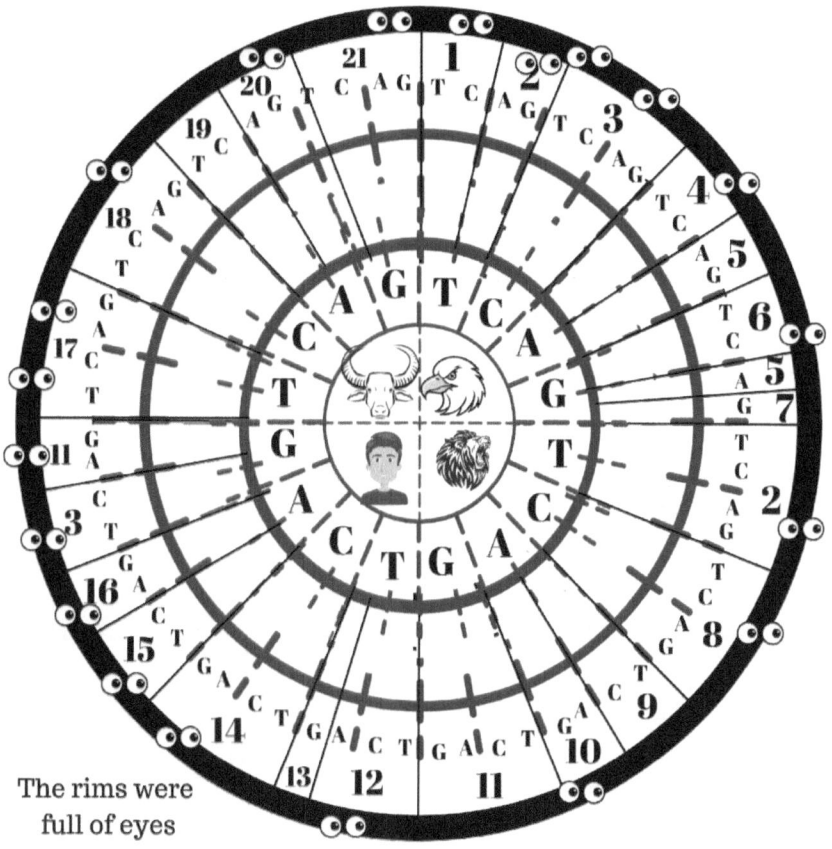

The rims were full of eyes

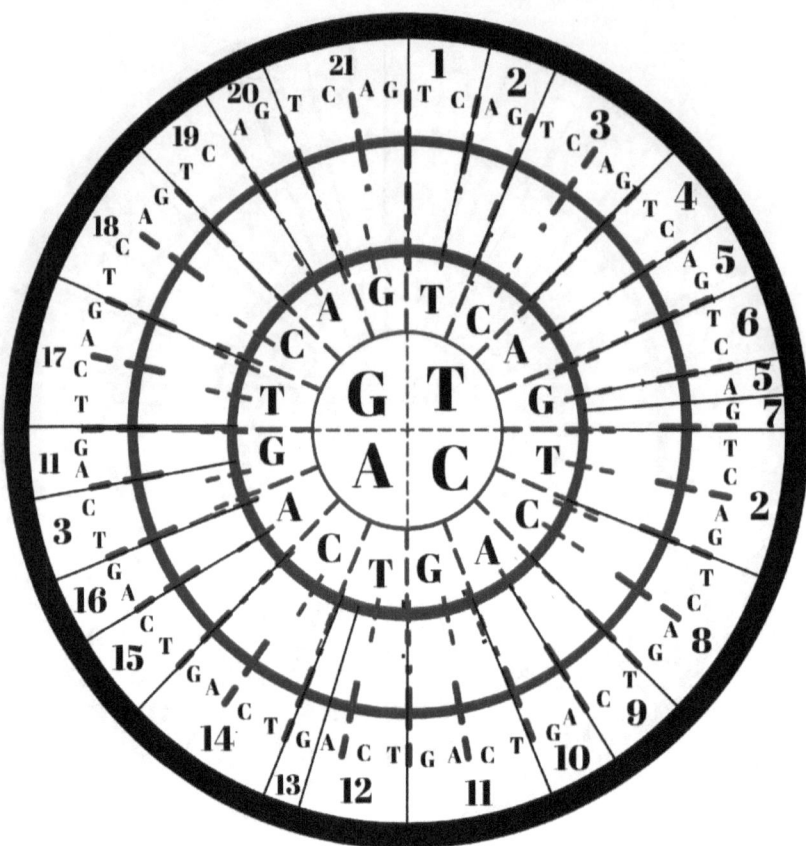

DNA Sequence Protein Combination Key

1	Phenylalanine
2	Leucine
3	Serine
4	Tyrosine
5	STOP
6	Cysteine
7	Tryptophan
8	Proline
9	Histidine
10	Glutamine
11	Arginine
12	Isoleucine
13	Methionine
14	Threonine
15	Asparagine
16	Lysine
17	Valine
18	Alanine
19	Aspartic Acid
20	Glutamic Acid
21	Glycine

DNA Sequencing Patterns and Rules

The body arranges each function of the body or an attribute or trait or characteristic of a person as a 12-letter DNA sequence based on the four bases of DNA namely Adenine [A], Cytocine [C], Thymine [T] and Guanine [G].

It derives at the number 12 letter word DNA sequence based on the letters of DNA that can combine to form a protein that is three letters of bases can form a protein. The body then look at four cycles and join these four cycles to form a word for that trait.

12 lettered DNA Sequence Name of any attribute or function

$$=$$

DNA Codon 1 = Protein Name

$$+$$

DNA Codon 2 = Protein Name

$$+$$

DNA Codon 3 = Protein Name

$$+$$

DNA Codon 4 = Protein Name

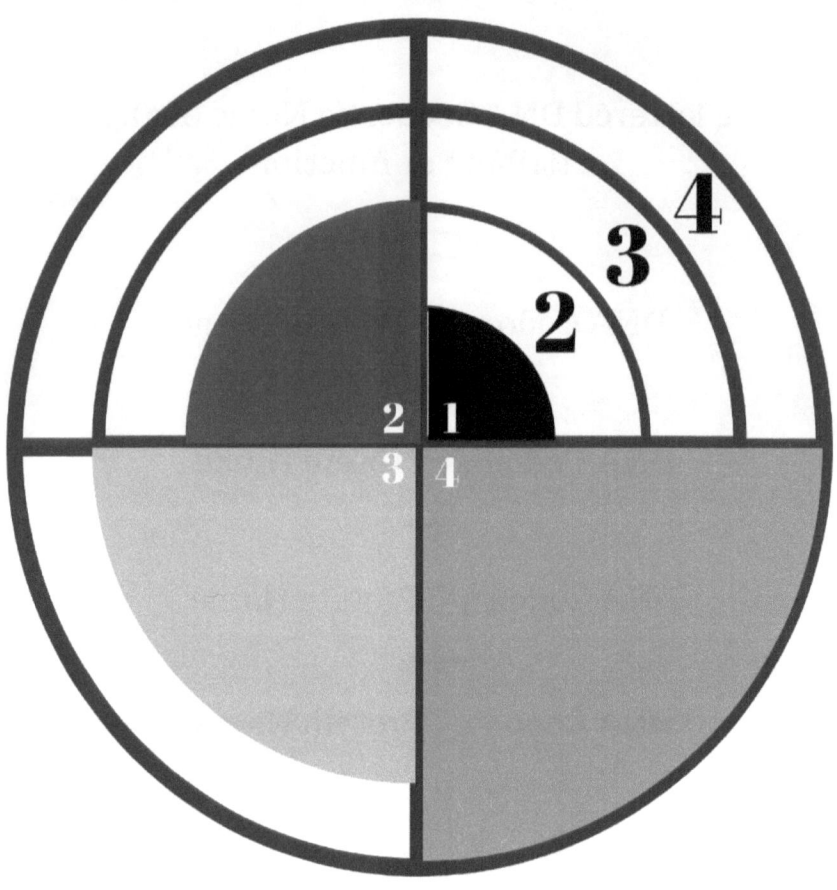

How the body determine the protein combination responsible for an attribute or function.
For example; DNA gene responsible for height is determined this way.
Height to the body in DNA sequence =
CTCCCGATCCCG

That means the Protein that can determine height is a combination of 4 proteins
3 possible combination x 4 cycles

=

12 letters
CTC +CCG+ATC+CCG

=

2+8+12+8

=

Leucine+Proline+Isoleucine+Proline

=

Is the combination of a protein that is responsible for height.

How the body determine the protein combination responsible for an attribute or function.
For example; DNA gene responsible for blue eyes is determined this way.
Blue eyes to the body in DNA sequence =
CTATACGTAGTA

That means the Protein that can determine blue eyes is a combination of 4 proteins
3 possible combination x 4 cycles

=

12

CTA +TAC+GTA+GTA

=

2+4+17+17

=

Leucine+Tyrosine+Valine+Valine

=

Is the combination of a protein that is responsible for blue eyes.

CHAPTER SIX

Now let us find out the protein combinations represented by the twelve letter DNA sequencing name. The body uses four seasons to denote a full complete cycle. Just like the seasons in nature, the body gives names to every function based on four codons each of three as only three letters of bases can represent a protein. We will use the wheel within a wheel to find out the protein representations.

It is ideal to bring that wheel here again.

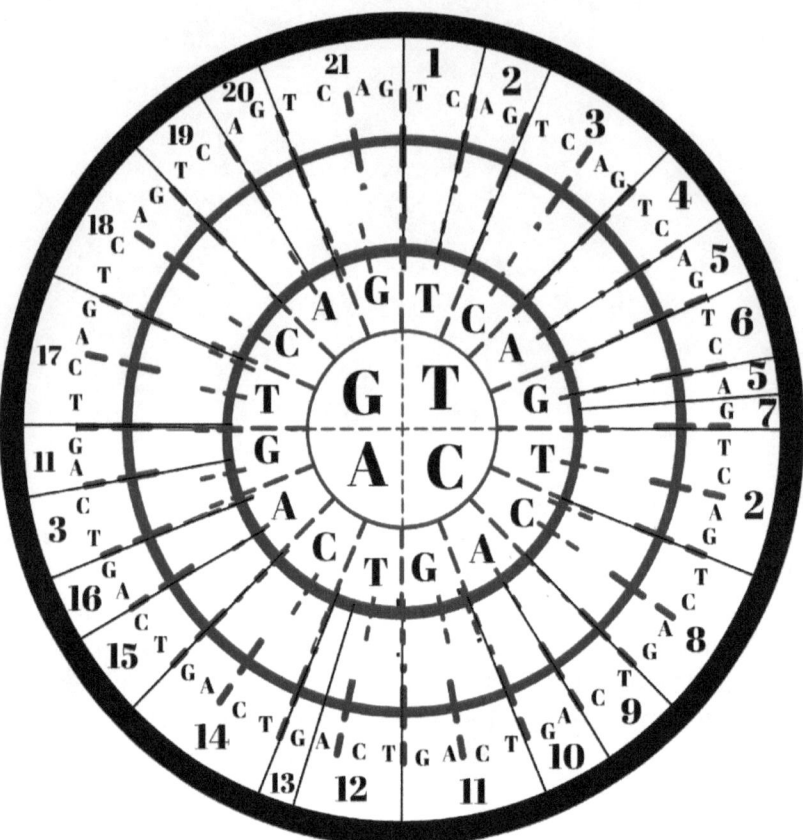

DNA Sequence Protein Combination Key

1	Phenylalanine
2	Leucine
3	Serine
4	Tyrosine
5	STOP
6	Cysteine
7	Tryptophan
8	Proline
9	Histidine
10	Glutamine
11	Arginine
12	Isoleucine
13	Methionine
14	Threonine
15	Asparagine
16	Lysine
17	Valine
18	Alanine
19	Aspartic Acid
20	Glutamic Acid
21	Glycine

Every three letters of the bases namely, Cytosine   C, Adenine A, Guanine G, and Thymine T will spell equivalent protein.

There are twenty amino acids.
Phenylalanine is represented by the number 1 on the wheel above.
Leucine is 2
Serine is 3
Tyrosine is 4
STOP is 5
Cysteine is 6
Tryptophan is 7
Proline is 8
Histidine is 9
Glutamine is 10

Arginine is 11
Isoleucine is 12
Methionine is 13
Threonine is 14
Asparagine is 15
Lysine is 16
Valine is 17
Alanine is 18
Aspartic Acid is 19
Glutamic Acid is 20
Glycine is 21

Now let us convert the twelve letter DNA sequence name to its protein forms using the wheel and the above category of protein.

Recap from the beginning.

Therefore, I can say that the female DNA sequence will start as follows.
Female left-hand thumb + Female left hand index finger + Female left hand middle finger + Female left hand ring finger + Female left hand little finger.

CTCTCTCTCTCC + GTAGTCGCCTCC + GTACCTATATCC + GTGTCCTAGACC + GTGTCTATGTCC

= female left hand fingers DNA sequence

This is equals to:
CTCTCTCTCTCCGTAGTCGCCTCCGTACCTATATCCGT GTCCTAGACCGTGTCTATGTCC.

Now let us convert this start of the female DNA sequence into its protein equivalent.

Female left-hand thumb = *CTCTCTCTCTCC* =*CTC +TCT+ CTC+TCC=2+3+2+3=leucine + serine + leucine*

+ serine

Female left hand index finger = *GTAGTCGCCTCC=GTA+*
GTC+GCC+TCC=17+17+18+3=valine + valine +
alanine + serine

Female left hand middle finger = *GTACCTATATCC =*
GTA+CCT+ATA+TCC = 17+8+12+3 = valine + proline
+ isoleucine + serine
Female left hand ring finger = *GTGTCCTAGACC =*
GTG+TCC+TAG+ACC = 17+3+5+14 = valine + serine
+ STOP+ threonine
Female left hand little finger = *GTGTCTATGTCC*
=GTG+TCT+ATG+TCC = 17+3+13+3 = valine + serine
+ Methionine + serine

Four possible START of a DNA sequence for a female are:
a] AAC =15=Asparagine
b] CAA = 10 = Glutamine
c] ACC = 14 = Threonine
d] TAC = 4 = Tyrosine

CHAPTER SEVEN

Ultimate recipe to create a female.
Therefore, this is the recipe for creating a female.
You can start with any of these.

Opening ingredients.
Asparagine or glutamine, threonine, or tyrosine

Add ingredients for the left-hand thumb.
add leucine and serine and leucine then serine.

Add ingredients for the index finger.
After that add valine then again add valine also add alanine
and serine.

Now add ingredients for the middle finger.
valine then add proline and isoleucine then add serine.

Now add ingredients for the ring finger.
valine then add serine then STOP and resume with adding
threonine.

Now add proteins for the little finger development.
Add valine then serine then Methionine and lastly add serine.

Now sit and relax while the proteins are at work making the female's left hand. You might want to start thinking about the name of this girl while the creation machine is at work. Or start working on the creation of a male. Here is the recipe.

Recap from previous chapters.
A male's starting DNA sequence is the starting DNA sequence from his left-hand thumb to the left-hand little finger. I explained above that all male DNA sequences for every part end with GA. Therefore, let us compile this DNA from the above information.

Male's starting DNA sequence.

Four possible START of a male DNA sequence are:
a] AAT = 3 = serine
b] CAT = 9 = histidine
c] ACT = 14= threonine
d] TAT = 4 = tyrosine

Therefore, depending on other factors I will explain in later chapters.

As such a male DNA sequence can be
AAT +
CTCTCTCTCTGACTCTGGCTCCGACTCTCCGTAGGACT
CTCCGATCGACTCCGAGATCGA.

This can be.
AATCTCTCTCTCTGACTCTGGCTCCGACTCTCCGTAGGA
CTCTCCGATCGACTCCGAGATCGA

Ther male DNA sequence can start with ACT.
That makes the DNA sequence be.
ACTCTCTCTCTCTGACTCTGGCTCCGACTCTCCGTAGGA
CTCTCCGATCGACTCCGAGATCGA

Male left hand thumb + Male left hand index finger + Male left hand middle finger + Male left hand ring finger + Male

left hand little finger
= *CTCTCTCTCTGA + CTCTGGCTCCGA +*
CTCTCCGTAGGA + CTCTCCGATCGA +
CTCCGAGATCGA
= *Male's left hand fingers DNA sequence*
=*CTC+TCT+CTC+TGA=2+3+2+5=leucine + serine +*
leucine + STOP
+*CTC+TGG+CTC+CGA=2+7+2+11 =leucine +*
tryptophan +leucine + arginine
+*CTC+TCC+GTA+GGA=2+3+7+21 = leucine + serine +*
tryptophan + glycine
+*CTC+TCC+GAT+CGA=2+3+19+ 11 =leucine + serine +*
aspartic acid + arginine
+*CTC+CGA+GAT+CGA=2+11+19+11 = leucine +*
arginine + aspartic acid + arginine

This is equal to.
CTCTCTCTCTGACTCTGGCTCCGACTCTCCGTAGGACT
CTCCGATCGACTCCGAGATCGA
= *leucine + serine + leucine + STOP+ leucine + tryptophan*
+*leucine + arginine leucine + serine + tryptophan + glycine*
+ *leucine + serine + aspartic acid + arginine leucine +*
serine + aspartic acid + arginine

The recipe for creating a male is the following.

Start by creating the male's left hand.
You will need the following as opening ingredients.
Serine, histidine, threonine, or tyrosine
For the left-hand thumb add the following.
leucine and serine add leucine then STOP.

For the left-hand index finger add the following.
leucine + tryptophan +leucine + arginine

Add the following for the middle fingers.
leucine + serine + tryptophan + glycine

For the ring finger add the following.
leucine + serine + aspartic acid + arginine

For the left-hand little finger add the following.
leucine + serine + aspartic acid + arginine

……TO BE CONTINUED IN VOLUME II…….

Further Reading.

How To Decode God, Creation, The Tree Of Life, Angels & Demons, The Devil, The Afterlife, The Underworld, The Brain, The Planets and The Universe.: The Definitive Guide.
https://play.google.com/store/books/details?id=1tLUEAAAQBAJ

As On Earth As In Heaven As It Is In Humans.: The Only True Explanation of The Use Of The Great Pyramid Of Giza. Debunked by David Gomadza.
https://play.google.com/store/books/details/David_Gomadza_As_On_Earth_As_In_Heaven_As_It_Is_In?id=I1rPEAAAQBAJ

The Time-Traveler: Back to the Assassination of Robert Kennedy
https://play.google.com/store/books/details/David_Gomadza_The_Time_Traveler?id=mTu9EAAAQBAJ

Encyclopedia of Decoding the Brain.: How To Decode the Brain. The Definite Guide.
https://play.google.com/store/books/details/David_Gomadza_Encyclopedia_of_Decoding_the_Brain?id=KcTPEAAAQBAJ

Brain Code. The Benchmark of Decoding the Brain.: One Against which all are Evaluated.

https://play.google.com/store/books/details/David_Gomadza_Brain_Code_The_Benchmark_of_Decoding?id=50a3EAAAQBAJ

THE GREATSHIFT: 2023 IS THE YEAR OF THE GREATSHIFT TO SUSTAINABLE ENERGY [PHASE ONE- ELECTRIC VEHICLES]

https://play.google.com/store/books/details/David_Gomadza_THE_GREATSHIFT?id=KH2xEAAAQBAJ

Proof of Aliens on Mars. A Must Read If You Are Serious About Mars.

https://play.google.com/store/books/details/David_Gomadza_Proof_of_Aliens_on_Mars_A_Must_Read?id=CUbHEAAAQBAJ

Tomorrow's World Order

https://play.google.com/store/books/details/David_Gomadza_Tomorrow_s_World_Order?id=VDauDwAAQBAJ

Visit our website

www.twofuture.world

If you can fund us donate
https://twofuture.world/donate

God's DNA Combination=
53 billion 600
Normal Human DNA Combination =
52 billion 200
Mine [David Gomadza]'s DNA
Combination pairs =
53 billion 600

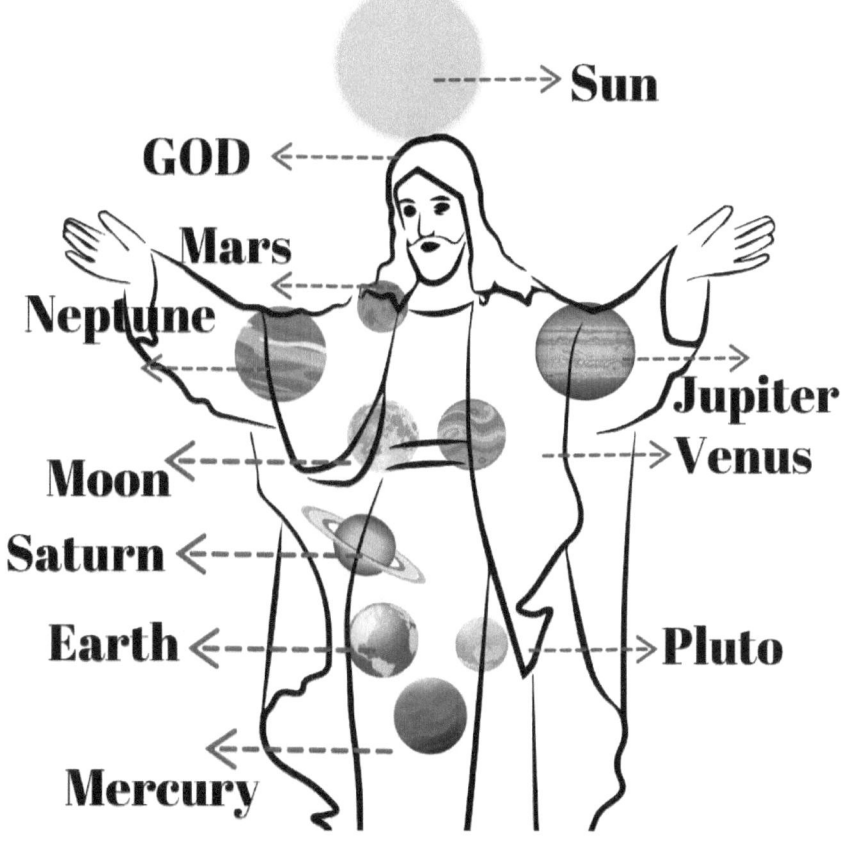

ABOUT THE AUTHOR

DAVID GOMADZA

I am the First Global President of The World
Visit www.twofuture.world
00447719210295
info@twofuture.world

Encyclopedia of Decoding DNA Sequence. A Definitive Guide.